R.E.I. Editions

All of our ebooks can be read on the following devices:

- Computers
- eReaders
- iOS
- Android
- Blackberries
- Windows
- Tablet
- Cell phone

French Academy

Anahata

The Fourth Chakra

ISBN: 978-2-37297-3670

Publication: February 2019
New updated edition: January 2023
Copyright © 2019 - 2023 R.E.I. Editions
www.rei-editions.com

Work plan

French Academy

Anahata
The Fourth Chakra

R.E.I. Editions

Book Index

The chakra system

The word Chakra, which comes from Sanskrit and means "wheel", is meant to indicate the seven basic energy centers in the human body. Chakras are centers of subtle psychic energy located along the spine. Each of these centers is connected, at the level of subtle energies, to the main ganglia of the nerves which branch off from the vertebral column. In addition, the chakras are related to the levels of consciousness, to the archetypal elements, to the phases inherent in the development of life, to the colors, which are closely linked to the chakras, because they are found outside our body, but inside the aura , or the electromagnetic field that surrounds each person, to sounds, body functions and much, much more. The Eastern doctrine that has spread knowledge of them in the Western world considers the Chakras as openings, gateways to the essence of the human body. The chakras are usually represented inside a lotus flower, with a variable number of open petals. The open petals represent the chakra in its full opening. On each petal is written one of the fifty letters of the Sanskrit alphabet, which are considered sacred letters, therefore, divine expression. Furthermore, each of them expresses a different activity of the human being, a different state, both manifest and still potential. Each chakra resonates on a different frequency which corresponds to the colors of the rainbow.

The seven main Chakras also correspond to the seven main glands of our endocrine system. Their main function is to absorb the Universal Energy, metabolize it, break it down and convey it along the energy channels up to the nervous system, feed the auras and release energy outside. Most everyone sees them as funnels, simultaneously swirling and flowing energy back and forth. Each of the seven centers has both an anterior (usually dominant) component and a posterior (usually less dominant) component, which are intimately connected, with the exception, however, of the first and seventh, which, however, are single.

From the second to the fifth, the anterior aspect relates to feelings and emotions, while the posterior aspect relates to the will. As regards the anterior and posterior sixth, and the seventh, the correlation is with the mind and reason. The first and seventh. they also have the very important connection function for the human being: being the most external Chakras of the energy channel, they have the characteristic of placing man in relation with the Universe on one side and with the Earth on the other. The perfect functioning of the energy system is synonymous with good health. There are many techniques to open the Chakras, including Reiki, which stands out for its peculiar sweetness and for the possibility of harmonizing any energy imbalances.

Each center oversees certain organs, and has particular functions on an emotional, psychic and spiritual level. Among the seven fundamental ones, there are precise affinities.

- The First with the Seventh: Basic Energy with Spirit Energy.
- The Second with the Sixth: Energy of feeling on a material level with Energy of feeling on an extrasensory level.
- The Third with the Fifth: Energy of the working mind and personal power with Energy of the higher mind and communication.
- The Fourth: bridge between the upper three and the lower three and alchemical forge of transformation.

Each Chakra is associated with a color, which corresponds to and derives from the frequency and vibration of the center itself. Furthermore, each Chakra corresponds to a mantra, the sound of a musical note and, in some cases, even a natural element, a planet or a zodiac sign. Because the chakra system is the primary processing center for every function of our being, blockage or energetic insufficiency in the chakras usually causes unrest in body, mind, or spirit. A defect in the flow of energy through a given chakra will cause a defect in the energy supplied to the connected parts of the physical body, as well as affect all levels of being. This is because an energy field is a Holistic entity; every part of it affects every other part. Essential oils are able to tune into specific chakras: their scent and their vibration gently put us in deep contact with our energy centers.

The massage with specific essential oils on the points corresponding to the chakras activates and balances their action, harmonizing and strengthening the entire body. Starting from the bottom they are:

- 1st = Muladhara
- 2nd = Swadhisthana
- 3rd = Manipura
- 4th = Anahata
- 5th = Vhishuddhi
- 6th = Ajna
- 7th = Sahasrara

Furthermore, each of the seven chakras comes to represent an important area of human psychic health, which we can briefly summarize as:

1. Survival
2. Sexuality
3. Strength
4. Love
5. Communication
6. Intuition
7. Cognition.

Metaphorically the chakras are related to the following archetypal elements:

1. Earth
2. Water
3. Fire
4. Air
5. Sound
6. Light
7. Thought

Anahata - The Fourth Chakra

The fourth chakra is also called the heart chakra, the heart center. Its symbol is the green lotus with twelve petals on which the twelve letters in Sanskrit stand out k, kh, g, gh, n (guttural), c, ch, j, jh, n (palatal), t, th (lingual), and is located in the region between the heart and the two nipples. Its geometric symbol is the double crossed triangle (six-pointed star). This chakra is located at the level of the cardiac plexus, behind the sternum, in the axis of the spinal cord and is the center of the entire Chakra system.

Due to its position, but also due to its function, it is the Chakra around which all the physical and energetic functions of man "revolve", it constitutes the transition and connection point between the three lower Chakras and the three upper ones. All the other Chakras therefore depend on this, since the heart is considered the seat of the spirit and the center from which all human emotions arise, especially love. In the Heart Chakra resides the divine spark that is within each of us, here is our enlightened nature, our Higher Self. This Chakra is considered the gateway to the soul, here feelings such as unconditional love, joy, inner peace, compassion, but also pain and emotional suffering originate. Every form of love originates here, whether it is love towards another person or the unconditional love that binds us to the universe. In it, up to the age of 12, antibodies would be produced, sent into the "subtle system" (a concept of Indian philosophy whose existence has no scientific confirmation, however) against external attacks on the body and psyche.

It develops during adolescence, from 12/13 years to the beginning of youth, towards 20/25 years.

Improper development or blockage of the heart chakra would cause feelings of insecurity.

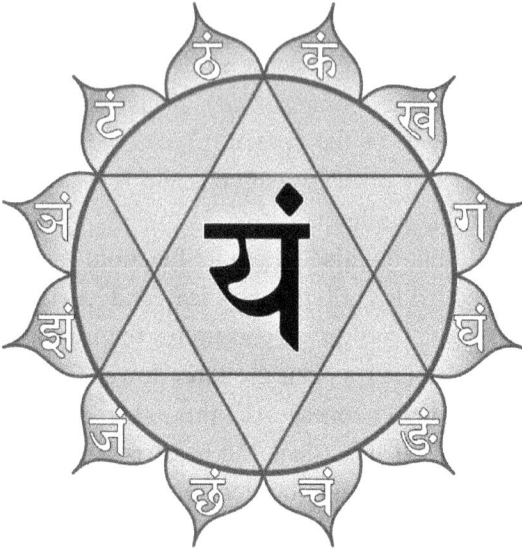

This chakra is associated with a healthy and dynamic personality, full of love and compassion and a love of family. It would close in case of conflicts in the family, abandonment, loss of a loved one.

This closure would over time affect the heart and lungs and cause pneumonia, asthma, heart disease. The pathologies connected to its imbalance are asthma, arterial hypertension, heart pathologies, pulmonary pathologies.

In the case of disharmonious functioning, on a physical level there may be symptoms in the chest, such as a sense of constriction, dyspnoea, arrhythmias, tachycardia, palpitations, asthma and so on, without however having objective evidence from clinical investigations. From a psychic and emotional point of view, we tend to love others only as a function of the acknowledgments and gratitude that they can give in return. If instead the Chakra is hypofunctional, on a physical level a malfunction of the diaphragm will be highlighted, with respiratory and cardiac problems, while from a psychic and emotional point of view there will be a tendency to express feelings of hatred and resentment, or of coldness, indifference or insensitivity.

It is through the harmonic activity of this Chakra that people are able to sympathize with everything that exists and to grasp its beauty and harmony. Indeed, the function of this energy center is that of the ability to express pure and unconditional love. The fourth Chakra is the center that allows the development and use of the ability to transform and heal oneself and others. The fourth is the middle chakra, the bridge that transforms and makes compatible the energies of the first three chakras, making them rise upwards, and of the last three, making them descend downwards. It allows you to love in a total sense and without conditions, everything and everyone. When the fourth chakra is open and vital, it makes it possible to relate to reality, seeing its entirety and accepting both its beauty and its negative aspects, enabling the person to give love without expecting anything in return.

In his posterior vision he represents the will of his own ego towards the external world, united with the divine will. It favors a harmonious vision of what surrounds the person and enables him to have positive attitudes regarding his own actions, seeing others as support for what he is doing. It is also the chakra through which all the energy you want to donate to others passes. Only if the fourth chakra is open and vital can healing energy be given. When it is closed or not harmonious, the person is hardly able to love and experience others, God or Destiny as you want to call them, in antithesis with themselves, as obstacles to their own fulfilment. And then we risk becoming aggressive and, instead of seeking help from others, we place ourselves in the classic condition of "me against everyone", instantly falling back into the disharmonious energy of the third chakra. Only if you consciously enter the energy of the fourth chakra, carrying and experiencing love and compassion, will you be able to give full meaning to your existence. The opening of the fourth chakra is therefore essential for the therapist: only by working with the heart can he, in fact, be placed in total availability towards others and in total sharing, while maintaining the necessary detachment. This chakra would also be associated with the thymus gland.

The thymus is a small lymphoid organ located under the breastbone that grows rapidly from birth to two years of age, then undergoes progressive atrophy and its activity is carried out by the immune system. It secretes hormone-like substances that increase the amount of white blood cells. In particular, it participates in the maturation process of T lymphocytes. The position of the thymus, near the heart, and the immune function are elements that signify a defensive role, the creation of a barrier which, if strengthened beyond a certain limit, can prevent love to enter the heart. In the absence of the thymus, the immune capacity does not develop and therefore there is no organic possibility of distinguishing the self from what is other than the self, the attacked from the aggressor. There is no possibility of balancing the opposites, of defending one's individuality. In this sense, the thymus guarantees the establishment of the maintenance of a harmonious balance between inside and outside, thus constituting the center of the individual's existence, its possibility of recognizing itself.

The correlated element is air represented by the smoky gray yantra made up of two triangles that intersect forming a six-pointed star, the central symbol of balance. The sense organ related to the anahata is the skin, seat of touch, while the organ of action are the genitals for the Shritattvacintamani, the hands and the faculty of grasping for some contemporary yoga masters.

The main feature of this chakra is mobility, so the concentration operated on the anahata makes what you want move.

The bijamantra «yam», i.e. the nasalized letter «ya», is that of the god Pavana, lord of the wind, represented as a smoky gray deity, with four arms, the goad in one hand, seated on a black antelope.

The heart distributes to the whole body, through the circulatory system, the blood that contains the oxygen fixed in the lungs during inspiration. It is here, like a sun that spreads its energy, a fire that, instead of burning, radiates its heat, warming and spreading life. Oxygen is, moreover, from an alchemical point of view, a solar element: fire can only burn in the presence of oxygen. Carbon dioxide returns to the heart and is released into the environment during exhalation.

It is thus a complete cycle, marked by the rhythmic repetition of systoles, a centrifugal force that sends blood to the body, and diastoles, a centripetal force that brings blood back to the heart. Two complementary phases, active and passive, birth (systole) and death (diastole), which repeat themselves continuously, cycle after cycle, and must be in perfect balance for the individual to exist.

The cardiac system is completely involuntary. The innervation of the heart, as well as that of the lungs (pulmonary and cardiac plexuses), comes, as far as the sympathetic nerve is concerned, from the band between the third cervical and fifth dorsal vertebra, involving the first, second and third cervical ganglion and the first thoracic ganglia; as regards the parasympathetic, from the vagus nerve that comes from the brainstem. The sympathetic system increases the frequency of the heartbeat and the force of contraction while, on the other hand, the parasympathetic has a function of decelerating the heartbeat. The so high position of the area of origin of these nerves may seem strange but, once again, it is enough to go back to the embryological development to explain this apparent discrepancy. In fact, in the very first stages of embryonic development, during the gastrulation process, a part of the mesoderm migrates up to the front of the pharyngeal membrane and unites with the homologous part of the opposite side (cardiac tube) forming the cardiac sketch, which only subsequently will place in a more ventral position (with the delimitation of the body of the embryo on the 22nd day). But the innervation will remain linked to the cervical metameres of its initial development. These metamers are also related to arm development. This link explains why arm-related pain can occur in heart-related conditions (for example, angina and heart attack). The lungs, similarly to the digestive system, put the inside in communication with the outside, they are a link between the individual and the cosmos, but for an energy that is more subtle than food, purer.

On the other hand, in more ancient stages of phylogeny, the respiratory and digestive functions were undifferentiated: «heavy» elements and «subtle» elements entered the organism together. Even today, the phylogenetically more primitive species (fish) maintain a single duct used both for feeding and for breathing (extroversion in the lateral walls of the digestive tract), while in other animals and in man a separation develops between the two functions : from the pharynx a "bag" differs which will become the lung which, therefore, is of common derivation with the digestive. In this case a possibility is evolving of extracting a more subtle material, of separating the light from the heavy.

The lung, in fact, captures the prana of the cosmos and "makes" it individual, puts the external "sun" (oxygen) in communication with the internal "sun" (heart).

The respiratory system also scans a complete cycle through each inhalation and exhalation which, in turn, are centripetal force and centrifugal force, birth and death, passivity and activity, brought together in a perfectly balanced rhythm.

But, unlike cardiac activity, respiratory activity is also voluntary, that is, it can be directed, modified, guided by consciousness. It is precisely to this thread (the possibility of voluntary control) that the yogi attaches himself to control, through breathing, the entire organism with its functions that are in themselves far from the domain of consciousness. Therefore, in this wheel there is also the balance of the conscious-unconscious duality, as foreseen by the cycle expressed by the number 12.

Therefore, also in the organs of the anahata chakra we find cycles characterized by complementarity of rhythms and functions which, in their balance, define the individuality of man.

Agni

In the Hindu religion, Agni is the god of fire, son of heaven and earth (Dyaus and Prthivi respectively), he is a Vedic deity who represents the forces of light; he is also an invincible warrior and is the lord of the cremation ground and the forest fire; of him is the "heat" generated in yoga practices. The main manifestation of him is "the fire that burns on the altar of sacrifices"; he burns the demons that threaten to destroy such sacrifices and is a mediator between gods and humans from whom the priests learn much about the afterlife. In this deity also persists the conception of "universal fire" which in man is identified in the heat of digestion; in fact, according to Ayurveda, Agni is the vital fire, which animates all biological processes, and represents the digestive metabolism.

Agni can manifest itself in three forms:

- Davagni
- Vavavagni
- Jatharagni (or Vrika).

The number 7 is related to Agni; in fact, 7 are the mothers, the sisters and the rays from which he is surrounded; he has the traits of an aquatic divinity and, in fact, is called "the one who wears the sea" and "the one who vivifies the seed in the water".

He is depicted in the form of a red man with two heads, four arms and three legs, dark eyes and flames coming out of his mouth, always riding a ram; in fact, from Agni derives the zodiacal sign of Aries, which is precisely a sign of fire. In his hands she holds the tools to rekindle the fire and the spoon for sacrifices.

According to other representations, his appearance is characterized by seven tongues and fiery hair or by a golden body, powerful teeth, a thousand horns and a thousand eyes.

How to activate the 4th chakra

- Open up to the beauty of nature, immerse yourself above all in green landscapes, such as woods or lush meadows.
- Treat yourself well, get regular massages or follow an Ayurvedic cure.
- Wear green clothing or decorate the house with this color, also place many plants in various corners of the house.
- Look after your relationships with your partner, family and friends. Make them solid and loving.
- Also have a spontaneously affectionate attitude towards your pets and your plants.
- Listen to sunny and joyful music, such as Mozart, Bach, Haydn.
- The vowel "A" stimulates this chakra. Sit down, relax, inhale and vibrate the "A" as you exhale. Repeat the exercise for 5 minutes.
- Learn shiatsu or Reiki.
- Essential oils: rose, jasmine, vanilla and tarragon stimulate the heart chakra.
- Precious stones: instinctively choose one of these stones, emerald, topaz, chrysoprase, green tourmaline, malachite, green spinel, jade.

Color of the fourth chakra

Green is the color of the second chakra.

The energy of the Heart Chakra is associated with the vibration of the color green, which symbolizes balance, compassion and harmony and conveys love for nature. It is the color that represents the union between terrestrial and celestial nature.

In the light spectrum, green is located in the center between cold and warm colors: it represents their synthesis and therefore performs a function of balance.

It is the therapeutic color par excellence, neither hot nor cold it has powerful rebalancing properties.

Those who love greenery have strong self-control and their strong character leads them to impose themselves on others. He is very routine, so he doesn't like changes and novelties, he defines himself as conservative and insecure in some ways. On the other hand, those who do not love greenery are people who set high expectations and are therefore often dissatisfied and suffocated. As we have guessed, chromotherapy suggests combining green with calm and inner peace. Indeed, the green palette refers to the concepts of money, destiny, luck and bad luck, hope, envy, health and energy.

In various parts of the world, green has different meanings. It is the typical color of Ireland, where it symbolizes the Celts, in China it indicates the betrayed husband, in Japan, eternal life and youth, while in India, harmony. Basically, however, as has been said, green is a symbol of tranquility, peace, hope, fertility and abundance.

Color is not just a chromatic mixture, but a set of sensations, ideas and thoughts that are evoked. A curiosity concerns the ancient caves, in which green does not appear because it is the color of vegetation and nature, therefore excluded. Centuries later, the Greeks left evidence of a very varied chromatic lexicon, where our color still does not appear, in favor of white, black and a vast range of reds. Not even Homer, poet par excellence in the popular imagination, ever mentioned green: for the ancients it was a mere pale shade that faded, weak and insignificant, among other colors. Only at the time of Pericles, in the fifth century BC, green finds space in the language: it is defined as prasinós, "leek", without attention to the different nuances.

However, the situation is very different among the Egyptians, where color was already used 4000 years ago with positive evocative meanings: the color of nature, vegetation and papyrus, it was the symbol of regeneration, associated with the supreme god Ptah, the Creator who ordered the great primordial Chaos and the world dominated by waters. Furthermore, even the god Osiris was called "The Great Green", that is the god who is reborn after death, therefore stones and objects in shades of green were auspicious.

The situation of the Latins is still different, who unlike the Greeks never had problems pronouncing the term viridis, hence our "green". For a long time it was considered a "barbaric" color, due to the color of the clothes that were dyed in this way. However, it was a color more strictly limited to women's clothing. In Rome, however, even newborns were wrapped in greenery, as a symbol of good luck, and women looking for a husband in the Middle Ages were dressed with the same intention, waiting for the happy event. The most common saying associated with this color is hope green. It is no coincidence that when faced with a natural expanse, where green is predominant, the feeling we have is precisely that of serenity and peace, rather than sadness. The color of the plant world is in fact always attributed to a positive rather than a negative sphere: emerald green represents relaxation and is useful for reducing mental stress and slowing down brain activity. In fact, its calming action works on the nervous system and stimulates lucidity and logic, making you more reflective. Green is among the recommended colors during a move and moments of transition, such as moving house, job or life changes, because it facilitates rooting.

Green not only gives a calming effect, but also instills a sense of justice and greatness of mind.

One of the benefits of the color green is unexpected, and concerns the emotional-psychological sphere: using this color on a white sheet, coloring, drawing abstract or precise shapes or writing relieves the load of anxiety and stress. It is no coincidence that when you have to make a decision of a certain importance, we advise you to surround yourself - in addition to white paper and a green marker - with objects of this colour, in the shade you prefer; the important thing is that they are always within sight, because they stimulate perseverance, which is needed in abundance in these situations.

- From a physiological point of view it promotes the general well-being of the organism, increases its vitality and restores the balance of its functions.
- It is used for the treatment of stress, anxiety, hyperactivity, headaches and some forms of insomnia.
- It is also effective in bulimia and in all psychosomatic forms that affect the gastrointestinal tract.
- It is also a powerful germicide and antibacterial.
- It has a positive effect on asthma, cough, joint inflammation, burns, bronchial diseases and the like.
- Detoxifies and decongests the body.
- It is very useful in case of headaches, neuralgia and fevers.

Effects on the psyche: calms, relaxes, eliminates tension, increases awareness, stimulates the eyes and enhances good mood. With the green color we obtain a harmony of the body. It represents the phlegmatic temperament. It is the color of concentration and guarantees precise control, exact analysis, coherent logic, good ability to record and remember. Green promotes harmony as it has a calming influence on the nervous system.

The desire for green fields and trees that one feels after a period spent among the gray pebbles and red bricks of the cities represents the instinctive yearning for the invigorating color of nature, which gives calm and refreshment.

Essential oils associated with the fourth chakra

Cypress, rose, lemon balm, neroli, verbena, pine, geranium, lavender, vanilla, lotus, myrtle activate the fourth chakra.

Mix each individual essential oil with a carrier oil, such as jojoba or almond oil, in the ratio of 2 drops per tablespoon of carrier oil, then 2 drops per 10 mL of carrier. Since this is a "vibrational treatment", a very diluted mixture will have a deeper and more marked action. Massage the chakra you want to work on with the blend containing the chosen essential oil. Use a few drops and apply them slowly with your fingertips and in a clockwise circular motion. While massaging the Chakra, focus on the result you want to achieve, visualizing the harmonic energy of the oil as it opens and rebalances the chakra. After the treatment, lie down and relax for a while, allowing the Chakra to rebalance itself. Breathe deeply and slowly, trying to clear and empty your mind as much as possible.

As an alternative to the massage, add a few drops of the essential oil chosen for the treatment to the essence diffuser. Concentrate and focus on your therapeutic intention, visualize the aromatherapy energy of the essential oil, open and rebalance the chakra. Relax for at least half an hour.

Cypress

Cypress essential oil is a very fragrant yellow-green oil. It has a rather sweet, balsamic smell with woody notes. Its beneficial properties are many. It has healing properties against hemorrhoids, capillary fragility, edema and rheumatism. It is beneficial for those suffering from bronchitis, cough and whooping cough. Cypress oil also has antiseptic and antispasmodic properties. And it's also a valid help against oily hair, acne and excessive sweat. It is ideal for those suffering from cellulite and water retention. Its healing properties can be exploited in moments of loss of space and order on a physical and psychic level. Cypress essence helps to restore the original shape, order or structure.

- Physical properties: cypress can be used for the following problems: cellulite, acne, couperose, hemorrhoids, varicose veins. Cypress prevents pollen allergies and gives relief in case of cough (also by combining it with cedar essential oil). In winter it is ideal as a home fragrance, because it prevents the negative effects of dry air.

- Psychic properties: In case of emotional stress it helps to regain strength in the psyche and body and restores understanding and inner structure. It also increases concentration and serenity, especially in distracted people. The application is recommended with a few drops of cypress in the base oil for back massage.

- 1 kg of essential oil is obtained from 70 kg of cypress branches.

In the Christian context, the cypress, together with the palm, the cedar and the olive tree, is considered one of the four woods with which the cross of Jesus was built.

• Antidepressant

As an antidepressant, if inhaled it has a general balancing action on the nervous system, softens changes and helps to overcome depression, which derives from the loss of loved ones and the end of a love story. Vaporized at home, 1-2 drops per square meter of the room, it can help overcome moments of stress or slight and momentary mental exhaustion.

• Invigorating bath

As a toning bath, pour 10 drops into the tub water, emulsify by shaking the water vigorously, then immerse yourself for 10 minutes to take advantage of the decongestant action for the circulatory and lymphatic systems. If you prefer the shower, pour 4 or 5 drops onto a wet sponge glove, possibly diluted in a little neutral liquid detergent, and rub in for at least 5 minutes.

- **Contraindications**

The internal use of the essential oil is not recommended during pregnancy, breastfeeding and hyperestrogenic women. Cypress essence is very powerful and should be used in small quantities.

Rose

The rose, a flower with exceptional properties, is an extraordinary rebalancing agent capable of strengthening the nervous system, promoting digestion and reawakening sexuality. Spring stress, which occurs after months of work, affects the health of the body, absorbing our energies and causing a lowering of the immune system. Rose essential oil reduces anxiety attacks, the constant feeling of tension and agitation generated by stress and the consequent somatic manifestations. Known for its numerous properties, it carries out a balancing, soothing and harmonizing action, useful for self-esteem and against anxiety and wrinkles. The rose is the archetype of the flower and the symbol of both profane and divine love. Known for more than 3,000 years, ancient civilizations used it as a main ingredient in the manufacture of perfumes and cosmetics along with other essential oils.

The Arabs and Berbers of Morocco have been distilling and producing rose water since the 1st century BC. C and used the infusion of its leaves for the anti-stress, tonic and antiseptic properties.

- The rose is one of the most difficult essences to distill, because it takes 4 to 5 tons of petals to obtain 1 kg of essential oil. In a drop of rose essential oil there is therefore the fragrance of about 30 roses; this low yield unfortunately justifies the high price of its essential oil. Rose essential oil is extracted from the Rosa damascena botanical species. Given the high costs of rose essential oil, there is no shortage of already diluted solutions on the market.

The harvest begins from mid-May to mid-June, at 4 in the morning and ends at 9; after this time, in fact, it becomes too hot, so the subtle volatile parts of the rose would be partially lost.

Rose essential oil is one of those essential oils which, at room temperature, gels; otherwise, when heated, it returns to a liquid state. This also determines the evidence of the genuineness of the real rose essential oil.

- **Harmonizing**

As a harmonizer, when inhaled, it opens and strengthens the heart. Rose essential oil relaxes the soul and activates the disposition for tenderness and love, as it develops patience, devotion and self-esteem. Gives joy and banishes negative thoughts, balancing negative emotions caused by anger, jealousy and stress. The scent of the essence is a wonderful psychological and physical support during pregnancy: excellent for accompanying women during childbirth and welcoming the new arrival with sweetness and love. In menopause it helps to soothe sadness and depression. In case of nervous depression, take 2 drops of rose essence twice a day.

- **Balancing of the female hormonal system**

If massaged on the stomach, it calms spasms in case of menstrual pain and stops bleeding. Indicated in disorders related to hormonal imbalances, anxiety and irritability that characterize premenstrual syndrome and menopause. To stimulate liver function, dilute 2 drops in 1 tablespoon of sweet almond oil and gently massage the liver area for a few minutes without pressing, just making a light circular rubbing to let the oil penetrate.

- **Stress reliever**

As an anti-stress, pour 4 drops of rose essential oil diluted in a tablespoon of jojoba oil and apply to the center of the forehead, under the chin and around the navel, with a circular message repeated three times: here is an excellent strategy to combat the stress. To complete and amplify the relaxing effect of the message, you can drink a cup of rose tea.

As a tonic against sexual asthenia, useful for a couple's massage or for a relaxing bath with an aphrodisiac effect; it is the oil of love and eroticism, because it enhances inner beauty and mitigates conflicts by instilling peace and happiness.

Prepare a massage oil by diluting 2 drops of rose essential oil and 2 drops of jasmine in 2 tablespoons of sweet almond oil.

- **Bath**

As an aromatherapy bath, pouring 10 drops of rose essential oil or, for an even more relaxing effect, 3 drops each of rose, ylang-ylang and sandalwood essential oils added to hot tub water will ease anxiety, tension and stress. and will promote night rest.

- **Contraindications**

At the recommended doses, it has no contraindications. Not suitable for children under 3 years of age, pregnant or breastfeeding women.

Melissa

The leaves of melissa, rich in essential oil, which gives the plant a pleasant aroma and the taste of lemon, are used in states of anxiety with somatizations affecting the gastrointestinal system. Due to its antispasmodic, anti-inflammatory and carminative action, it is indicated in case of menstrual pain, neuralgia, digestive disorders, nausea, flatulence, abdominal cramps and colitis. This plant is also used in the treatment of headaches, when it is caused by nervous tension, thanks to the presence of the essential oil (0.5%) which acts as a calmer on the nervous system, and relaxing on the muscles. Its use is particularly indicated, therefore, in the presence of a picture of general irritability, insomnia caused by excessive tiredness, nervousness, premenstrual syndrome, and tachycardia on a functional basis.

- It takes 10,000 kg of Melissa to have just 1 liter of oil.

In aromatherapy, lemon balm is considered a real panacea for the mind. It is counted among the natural remedies for anxiety, a panacea against stress and various psychosomatic disorders, emotional shocks and physical traumas, after serious news, as a mood support. It acts quickly and for this reason it is considered a natural anxiolytic. Mitigate strong emotions and compensate for excesses. In case of frequent panic attacks, pour a few drops of essence into the aroma diffuser, its pleasant scent carries out a balancing, refreshing and invigorating action on the environment. It is a very powerful essential oil, of great benefit on the heart chakra and, in fact, it is very suitable for those suffering from heart disease; its solar energy tones the heart, regulates blood pressure, calms states of anxiety and stress and therefore their effects on the circulatory system.

As a sedative it exerts a relaxing action on the nervous system, calms tension and anxiety and all the manifestations of a psychosomatic nature connected to these conditions, such as palpitations, headache, gastritis.

- **Insomnia**

For insomnia, 2 drops in a carrier oil massage into temples and abdomen to calm, relax and induce sleep. Then put 7-8 drops of Melissa essential oil in an essence burner or in a humidifier designed for essences and place it in the chamber.

- **Migraine**

For migraine, put 6 drops of Melissa essential oil in 200 ml of cold water and apply compresses to the forehead with a soaked cloth. While doing the poultices, remain lying down until the discomfort passes.

- **Contraindications**

Melissa has some side effects.

Its use is not recommended in case of therapies based on thyroid hormones, it could lead to paradoxical effects with states of agitation. Not suitable for children under 3 years of age, pregnant or breastfeeding women. Care must be taken, as it is one of the most frequently adulterated oils.

Real Melissa oil is very expensive, and is often replaced with other oils with a similar aroma, such as lemongrass or lemon verbena. These oils have their own properties, which are very valid, but they are certainly not the same as Melissa, so it is important to buy the oil only from trusted suppliers who can guarantee that this is really the oil you need.

Neroli

Neroli essential oil is a vegetable oil produced by distillation of bitter orange blossoms. Its scent resembles that of bergamot. Sweet scent of the flower and bitter taste of the fruit characterize the bitter variety of orange. The essential oil of neroli is extracted from the flowers of the bitter orange which differs from the sweet variety due to its longer thorns, their darker colour, the more intense aroma of the leaves and flowers, the more colored and rougher skin of the fruit, but above all for the particular bitter taste of the pulp. This double aspect is also found in love and for this reason neroli essential oil has always been its symbol. Known for its numerous properties, it has a calming, rebalancing and regenerating action, useful against stress and menstrual pain.

The scent of neroli essential oil is sweet, honeyed, with slightly metallic and spicy facets. It is a less floral scent than that of the classic orange blossom.

Neroli is one of the expensive essential oils, because it takes a ton of orange blossom to make a liter of essence. Neroli is one of the few essential oils that has been scientifically proven to increase the production of serotonin in the brain. Serotonin is an important neurotransmitter and is capable of altering mood; in fact, when it is present at high levels, it increases our feeling of serenity and well-being.

Neroli essential oil is indicated after mental fatigue and psychic tension, against fear, anxiety disorders, depression and calms thoughts in times of confusion. Bring peace to your heart, cheerfulness and comforting optimism. In afflictions it helps us to lighten its burden. It strengthens us in situations where we see no way out. It exerts an effective calming action in case of emotional disturbances, nervousness, insomnia, hypertension, tachycardia, stress. It reconciles sleep and is very useful in case of overexcited children who fall asleep with difficulty. Apply 2 drops of neroli essential oil (diluted, on delicate skins, in a little almond oil) on the inner surface of the wrists and rub them vigorously against each other, while raising the arms upwards, to better inhale the aroma that is released, through deep breathing.

- **Emotional shocks**

In case of emotional shocks, fears, stress, dilute 3 drops of essential oil in a teaspoon of almond oil and massage a little on the central part of the sternum. In case of mild depression, insomnia, anxiety, take an aromatic bath by pouring 8 drops of neroli essential oil and 8 drops of lavender essential oil on 3 handfuls of unrefined sea salt; add the mix to the hot tub water. Alternatively, receive a massage on the whole back performed with flavored sesame oil in the following proportions: for 50 ml of vegetable oil add 6 drops of neroli essential oil, 5 drops of geranium essential oil and 5 drops of myrrh essential oil.

This essence is comparable to the "Rescue Remedy" in Dr. Bach flowers, as it helps us overcome fears, traumas, shocks and depressions.

• Relaxing bath

As a relaxing bath, mix 10 drops of neroli in the tub water, taking care to close the door and windows tightly to keep the vapors inside the bathroom and be able to breathe them.

• Contraindications

At the recommended doses, it has no contraindications. Keep out of the reach of children under 3 years of age.

Vervain

Known for its numerous properties, verbena essential oil is anti-inflammatory, febrifuge and calming, also useful for gastric functions and airway infections. It has antispasmodic activity, sedates spasms and pains of psychosomatic origin, acting as a normalizer and calming. Anti-inflammatory and febrifuge, thanks to its refreshing properties, it soothes joint inflammation and lowers fever. Antiseptic and disinfectant in case of upper respiratory tract infections. Calming, it is a mood rebalancing but also a tonic of the nervous system, it strengthens concentration and memory. Digestive and liver stimulant, it facilitates gastric functions and nutrient absorption.

The Romans considered verbena a propitiatory plant and it was used for the purification ceremonies of the altars and to accompany the activities of the ambassadors. Indeed, before leaving, these dignitaries were touched with branches of verbena collected in a sacred place on the Capitoline Hill to confer on them the powers of representation of the Roman state.

- **Invigorating bath**

As an invigorating bath, pour 15-20 drops of verbena essential oil into the bath water. To combat anxiety, stress and insomnia, before going to sleep enjoy a nice relaxing bath, adding 15-20 drops of oil to the tub water and remaining immersed for 20-30 minutes. This moment of relaxation will also help fight rheumatic pains and muscle spasms, because this essence tones and helps eliminate toxins.

- **Contraindications**

Verbena essential oil is not recommended for children under six years of age, it should not be used during pregnancy and breastfeeding. For the rest it does not present particular contraindications, but it is good not to expose yourself to the sun after using it, because it can give rise to photosensitivity phenomena, due to the presence of citral.

Pine tree

Scots pine essential oil is a general stimulant of the nervous system, adrenal glands, mucolytic, expectorant, antiseptic, lymphatic decongestant, antirheumatic, anti-inflammatory, deodorant, sexual tonic, hypertensive. The essence released by the Scots pine essential oil penetrates easily through the skin, where it performs its functions as a fluidifier, sedative of the cough and of the upper respiratory tract.

From the resin that tends to form on the trunk, the essence of turpentine is extracted by steam distillation, a transparent, amber liquid with a strong smell and an acrid, bitter taste, used for centuries for numerous therapeutic indications including bronchitis , rheumatism and skin affections.

Four methods of extracting turpentine are known, depending on which part of the tree is used to obtain it:

1. That of the resin, in which the amount of turpentine amounts to 25%, which is steamed out of pine exudate.
2. That of the wood, which can be extracted using solvents from the heartwood of the trunk left to ferment for about fifteen years.
3. That of dry branches or trunk, obtained by providing heat.
4. That of wood pulp, in the paper industry when the resinous portion is separated from the pulp.

Among the Assyrians he was considered the "guardian of life". In ancient times, pine needles were used by American Indians to fill mattresses to keep fleas and insects away.

• Invigorating

As a tonic it helps to feel immediately efficient upon awakening, indicated in cases of hypotension and heart failure. It is used to remove the sense of tiredness in people who are tired or under stress, in case of sleep disturbances or nervous exhaustion.

This essence stimulates the adrenal cortex which regulates the production of hormones in response to stress by the body, therefore, it is particularly effective for reinvigorating and toning.

Due to its stimulating action, the essential oil can help in the treatment of impotence, frigidity, in case of sexual disorders or decreased libido. Its peculiar balsamic and expectorant effects but above all the ability to tone the muscular system of the respiratory system.

• Contraindications

Pine essential oil is contraindicated in pregnancy and in high doses it can irritate the mucous membranes. Applied externally at high concentrations it can give rise to sensitization effects. It is advisable to avoid its external use if there are skin irritations.

As with any other essential oil, even for Scots pine it is advisable to consult an herbalist before using it, in order to fully and safely exploit its numerous benefits.

Geranium

In aromatherapy, geranium essential oil is used in case of acne, anxiety, depression, stress, insomnia and sore throat. Geranium essential oil has antibacterial, antidepressant, anti-inflammatory, antiseptic, astringent, diuretic, repellent and tonic properties. This makes it suitable for use on a variety of health and well-being issues.

It is also used to promote emotional stability, to relieve pain thanks to its pain-relieving properties, to stimulate the healing of burns and wounds thanks to its healing properties, to improve mood and to reduce inflammation. It is useful for performing leg massages to reactivate circulation.

Originally from South Africa, geranium was introduced into Europe in the 17th century by English and Dutch colonists, who, returning from the Indies, stopped with their ships at the Cape of Good Hope to get supplies. In our continent it has begun to be cultivated, especially in the Mediterranean area, which has a climate similar to that of its origin.

The oil that is extracted from the geranium, as soon as it is distilled, looks like a green liquid with a very delicate sweetish smell, which is then worked and mixed according to the needs or left in its pure state.

- **Rebalancing**

As a rebalancing, it is used in aromatherapy to increase imagination and intuition so as to be able to find solutions in tangled or difficult situations. It stimulates the will and desire to express yourself and to bring out what you feel deep down, it helps to become aware and balance the give-and-take. Very suitable for people who don't know what they want, it stimulates motivation in them. Attract to us all that is positive. It helps promote sleep and relaxation. You can apply a few drops on a handkerchief to place on the bedside table or keep close to the pillow, or give a neck and shoulder massage before going to sleep.

- **Invigorating**

As a tonic it is indicated in massages to reactivate blood circulation, to fight cellulite, and in the treatment, prevention or normalization of disorders that originate from a malfunction of the circulatory system, such as varicose veins, capillary fragility and couperose. Geranium essential oil is considered helpful in preventing and relieving wrinkles.
That's why it is used as an ingredient in anti-aging creams. You can add a single drop of geranium essential oil to the moisturizer you usually use for your face.

- **After Sun**

As after-sun, dilute 5 drops of Geranium essential oil, 5 of Chamomile and 1 of Peppermint in a spoonful of Jojoba Oil and add to the bath and/or rub before going to sleep.

- **Contraindications**

Geranium essential oil is considered safe, so there are no particular precautions to follow. It's important to remember that the improper use of essential oils can be harmful, so always rely on the advice of an herbalist.

Lavender

Originally from southern and western Europe, the Provençal one is the most famous; it was already a precious plant for the ancient Romans who put bunches of flowers in the water of the thermal baths.

The rather fragrant flowers are grouped in thin blue-violet spikes. Lavender was already used then as a base for refined perfumes and to prepare decoctions and infusions used for the beauty of skin and hair. In the more recent past we know that in every city or country house there was no wardrobe or chest of drawers that did not have sachets of lavender to perfume the linen and keep moths away.

This delicate custom is now making a comeback and reminds us of ancient traditions and sensations of cleanliness and care for the home.

The French chemist, Renè Maurice Gattefossé, who is credited with the invention of the term "aromatherapy" in 1928, and who contributed to the resurgence of interest in the use of essential oils for therapeutic purposes, had at his own expense, noted that the Lavender essential oil, which he was using for perfume blends, had remarkable ability to heal burn wounds. In fact, while he was working on perfumes he accidentally burned his arm and as a reaction he slipped it into the liquid closest to him. It so happened that that liquid was precisely lavender essential oil which made him heal from the burn in a very short time.

Lavender essential oil has both external and internal use. Combined with creams, or dropping a few drops into hot bath water, or even applied directly to the skin for massages, it helps purify fatty and impure epidermis, facilitates the healing of sores, abrasions and wounds, stimulates circulation, especially that of the scalp. The aroma emanating from lavender essential oil is relaxing and sedative and massaged on the back of the neck it seems to help keep lice away.

Lavender essential oil is one of the few oils in this family that can also be used pure, although it is always recommended to dilute it in water, creams or gels.

- As with many other essential oils, pregnant or nursing women should avoid using lavender essential oil.
- It is also recommended that patients with diabetes to stay away from lavender oil.
- It can also cause allergic reactions in people who have particularly sensitive skin.
- Some people may also experience nausea, vomiting and headaches due to using the wrong essential oil.
- Most importantly, lavender oil should never be ingested, but only applied topically or inhaled through means of aromatherapy or similar activities.
- Ingestion may cause serious health complications, characterized by blurred vision, difficulty breathing, burning eyes, vomiting and diarrhea.

• Contraindications

Lavender essential oil has no particular contraindications. However, always remember to use it by inhalation or in friction and, if in doubt, always consult your doctor before using it. In fact, it is good to remember that essential oil, although it is considered safe, could have some contraindications if used improperly or excessively. Therefore, the consultation of the doctor or herbalist must be requested.

Vanilla

The sensual and enveloping fragrance that distinguishes vanilla comes from this wonderful orchid native to Mexico. In particular from its fruits, called pods, from which the precious spice is extracted. It has excellent aromatherapy properties: it is relaxing, antidepressant, rebalancing, calming, therefore excellent for combating stress and insomnia.

Vanilla is also a natural antioxidant, fights free radicals and is a good antiseptic.

- It is said to be a powerful stimulant of the sexual sphere; it is, in fact, known for its aphrodisiac properties.

With vanilla essential oil you can prepare deodorants that neutralize bad smells, without inhibiting sweating, but highlighting the person's smell. Great for perfuming face blends, vanilla essential oil is good for all skin types because it's a balancer. Vanilla has an intense but at the same time pleasant aroma and is also used in aromatherapy. Vanilla is grown in all tropical countries but the most prized and best known is Bourbon vanilla from Madagascar.

Aphrodisiac, in moments of disappointment and discouragement, for those who fear losing control. It relaxes and sweetens any conflict. Eliminate frustrations, fear and a sense of abandonment. Arouses a feeling of well-being and relaxation, and is an excellent antidepressant. Make massages by putting 10 drops of vanilla essential oil in 2 tablespoons of vegetable oil. Its aroma fights aggression, excitement and stress.

As an anti-stress, put 3 drops of vanilla essence on a handkerchief and breathe deeply the aroma or proceed with a relaxing massage by putting 10 drops of vanilla essential oil in 2 tablespoons of vegetable oil. You can also massage the temples and forehead with the previous mixture using 3 drops.

- **Contraindications**

Vanilla essential oil is generally well tolerated, non-irritating and non-sensitizing. For safety, however, before using it, always do a small test on the body, diluting two drops of essence in sweet almond oil or other vegetable oil and massage on a point at will. If nothing has appeared within a few hours, you can safely use vanilla. To be avoided in case of pregnancy or breastfeeding and in children under 3 years.

It is extensively adulterated.

Myrtle

The essential oil is obtained from the leaves and young twigs with the steam distillation method and a light orange colored liquid is obtained which gives off an intense sweet scent. The myrtle was consecrated to Venus because the goddess, after being born from the waters of the sea of Cyprus, had taken refuge in a myrtle wood, therefore the object of propitiatory offerings, during her sacrifices.

It was considered one of the symbolic plants of Rome, so much so that in the Forum there was an ancient altar consecrated to Venus Mirtea. Myrtle was a plant linked to beauty, but also to heroism. Greeks and Romans considered this plant the symbol of material joys, glory and happy love. For this reason, crowns were made for heroes and brides.

Christianity wanted to dedicate the myrtle to the happiness of newlyweds, for which it was used as a good omen in wedding parties. In fact, in the past young brides used a myrtle crown as a symbol of purity, hope and the beginning of a new life.

As a tonic, if inhaled it restores the inner smile, it helps to find solutions to get out of difficult situations and deeply negative experiences. Its perfume frees the breath, opens the chest and has a positive effect on the soul stressed by everyday thoughts. Myrtle is an excellent aid for hyperactive, insecure and stressed children from school life. In addition to stimulating profane love, this plant is a friend of the spirit, therefore also stimulating the 7th chakra.

Definitely useful for hypochondriacs, it relieves the fear of illness and gives a serene idea of death. Associated with helichrysum it helps to overcome a bad relationship with one's sexuality.

- **Contraindications**

There are no particular contraindications in taking myrtle, the only side effect could be skin allergies. Contraindicated in pregnancy, for children up to three years of age and in cases of severe hepatic and/or renal insufficiency. In high doses it can cause nausea, depression and headaches.

Himalayan flowers for the fourth chakra

Himalayan Flower Enhancers directly affect the various energy levels controlled by the Chakras, removing negative feelings and stimulating positive ones. The Himalayan Flower Enhancers were identified by Tanmaya in 1990, during a stay of several months in a Himalayan valley. The term Enhancers means catalysts, because the essences are not only remedies aimed at working on negative emotions and inner states but also favor very deep processes of energy rebalancing and spiritual development to bring to light qualities buried within the person. They can be taken pure alone or diluted together with Bach flowers or other flowers. Tanmaya's first preparations involved nine combinations, seven directly connected to the plexuses, better known by the Indian name of chakra plus a general catalyst and a flower particularly suitable for children; subsequently their number multiplied with the discovery of new flowers, suitable for modulating specific emotions.

They are Flowers with a very rapid and powerful effect, unlike Bach Flowers, which are among the slowest and most delicate; this power is sometimes very useful, other times it can represent a risk of excessive action. While Bach Flowers can be considered primarily emotional remedies, i.e. aimed at rebalancing human emotions, Himalayan Flowers, thanks to the nature of the soil on which they grow, essentially address the spiritual dimension of man, stimulating the need for prayer, of meditation and connection with the divine that dwells in him.

Himalayan floral essences are liquid extracts that contain the energy of the flower to be administered generally orally, and can also be used in bath water, sprayed on the body or in the environment, or combined with oil for massage.

Ecstasy

It fosters love, compassion, sincerity, a sense of truth, depth of feeling, a sense of expansion and universal togetherness, service and generosity.

Stimulates empathy with all living creatures, can solve situations of rigidity, contraction and bitterness, dissolves jealousy, lack of affection and psychic nutrition, hyper-criticism, distrust, irritability.

It helps to temper criticism, selfishness, attachment, jealousy, a sense of superiority, rationality and detachment. There are moments in life when we feel love for all people, for all things, life seems beautiful to us, the earth a beautiful place where nothing can go wrong. In this case our fourth chakra is working well, we are in empathy with the world and with life, full of love. Other times it is not like this: we do not feel love, either for human beings or for life, we are jealous, selfish, we attach ourselves to who or what gives us security, we do not like contact with people and we would like to be alone, close around the house and don't talk to anyone about our problems or theirs.

When the flow of energy into the fourth chakra is blocked, emotions become shriveled, withdrawn, cold, detached, and numb. Maybe we have suffered a pain, a loss, a sorrow, we are torn and in crisis, our partner has betrayed or abandoned us; we defend ourselves by closing ourselves off, hoping in this way never to suffer like this again.

But at a certain point we discover that this is not the case, that we are losing among the highest human qualities, those of love and hope.

Ecstasy fosters love, compassion, sincerity, a sense of truth, depth of feeling, a sense of expansion and universal love, service and generosity. Stimulates empathy with all living beings, reduces rigidity, contractions, bitterness, jealousy, lack of affection, hypercriticism, distrust and irritability. With Ecstasy the energy of the fourth chakra returns to flow and with it emotions and love, joy, openness, the courage to take risks, generosity, service to the world. The dosage of essences, pure or diluted, is two drops under the tongue several times a day.

Ecstasy is not recommended for those who already tend to be weak and impressionable, because this side of the character would be strengthened..

Californian flowers for the fourth chakra

The Californian Flowers extend the Bach Flowers.

Richard Kats and Patricia Kaminski, founders of the FES (Flower Essence Society), together with the work of other researchers have discovered more than 150 flowers since 1979. They work on more modern and current specific problems which at the time Bach lived did not they were so preponderant or they weren't talked about like today: anorexia and bulimia, sexual disorders, diseases deriving from environmental pollution. It is possible to create composite essences by combining Bach and Californian flowers, as well as essences from other flower therapy repertoires from other parts of the world. Californian flower remedies are prepared in the same simple way as Bach flowers, by placing wild flower corollas in a glass bowl filled with spring water and leaving them to infuse in the sun for a few hours. This liquid, very rich in vital force, is then filtered, diluted in brandy and used for the preparation of the so-called stock bottles (or concentrates).

The choice of essences, as with Bach flowers, is always personalized and in relation to the mood and emotions you want to rebalance. Once the remedy or remedies indicated for the personal problem have been chosen, two drops of each are poured into a small bottle with a 30 ml dropper, filled with natural mineral water and two teaspoons of brandy as a preservative.

The dosage is 4 drops 4 times a day, for a period of a few weeks or in any case until the symptoms improve or disappear.

Being a completely natural and non-toxic cure, they have no contraindications, do not cause side effects, can be combined without problems with both traditional and homeopathic medicines (of which they are considered complementary) or other flower therapy remedies.

Bleeding Hearth

This is the essence for those who are to learn the spiritual lesson of love and freedom.

It is for those who completely invest their feelings in another person and when the latter is no longer present, they find themselves flooded with anguish. Tendency to create relationships based on fear, affective possessiveness, or mutual dependence, inability to love unconditionally. Anxiety about broken relationships or the death of one's partner when one lived in symbiosis. This intense need to bond is often experienced by the partner as an emotional dependence, provoking the need for detachment, since such a dependent relationship is deprived of true freedom and balanced exchange. This essence provides the energetic support to accept the end of a relationship or the loss of a loved one.

It favors the opening of the heart chakra thus giving the possibility to let a feeling flow freely and totally, free and unconditionally.

The loved one is no longer experienced as a property that one fears losing and thus one is freed from affective and emotional dependence.

These are individuals who find themselves prisoners of symbiotic emotional ties, attachments and ties from which they cannot, nor are they able to separate, even if they want to. They have dependent and insecure personalities in their emotional bonds, but they are also very possessive.

Many of these people can have an egocentric and excessively self-centered character and tend to discriminate a lot about what is their own and what is other people's. The central problem of these subjects is the pathological nature of the relationships they establish and the poor ability to tolerate frustration. The essence helps to separate from possessive relationships, gives freedom in love, allows the partner to grow in freedom.

It gives security and disinterest, acceptance and detachment. It helps to process and deal with the painful experience of the first love disappointments.

It gives the ability to learn not to be emotionally dependent on others.

With the Bleeding Heart flower essence the individual learns to fill himself from within with strong spiritual energies, so that the ability to love the other is based on the ability to respect and feed the ego.

Borage

For affective depressions.

Who has lived a great pain of heart and now feels the oppression in the chest, a weight in the heart due to pains of love. Brings back serenity, good mood and will to live, soothes pain.

Gives the courage to carry on in difficult situations having self-confidence (once the plant was called Corago, instead of Borago, referring precisely to the courage associated with it).

When our heart becomes too thinking and sad, we get discouraged, we get discouraged.

This essence helps to regain lightness of heart, to feel vivacity and lightness, filling the person with energy and optimism. It is also useful in midlife crises when there is a deep, unexpressed angst and awe at what one has failed to achieve. Useful to soothe the pain caused by an abortion. In menopause when the end of the period causes anguish because one can no longer conceive or when one cannot find a partner. In mourning, to overcome the pain of feelings that oppress the heart, due to the death or impending death of the loved one. Dissipates pessimism, melancholy and all depressive states resulting from exhausting affective experiences. Relieves emotional and mental tensions by restoring good mood, hope and the will to live. It also acts as a purifier of toxins produced by negative moods.

The lesson to be learned is to face the sufferings and misfortunes of life with strength and courage.

Borage flower essence helps the heart to experience this vivacity and lightness, filling the individual with energy, optimism and enthusiasm, it is an excellent all-purpose balm and tonic to be used in many compounds, when the person needs to lift and of encouragement.

Oregon Grape

The person feels persecuted is always on the defensive and others isolate him for his attitudes. This leads him into a state of solitude.

Oregon Grape is indicated for people full of paranoia; they see hostility and disloyalty in the world and in the people around them.

These patterns were learned in childhood from family or upbringing and have not been remedied; on the contrary, they rot in the soul and continue to infect all human relationships and social situations. Unfortunately, the individual oppressed by this state of paranoia creates the very reality that he projects, since those who are treated in a hostile or distrustful manner generally react by adopting the same attitude.

Oregon Grape has many uses, but is best suited for the tension and malice that predominate in many city environments. With Oregon Grape the individual learns to break the patterns of distrust that he has behind him. He realizes that he can, instead, pick up on the positive intentions of others and create situations that engender goodness and loving understanding.

Trillium

For those who, rich or poor, have unbridled ambition and think that happiness can only be accessed through material goods. Thus he falls back into forms of greed and lust for power.

Trillium flower essence is a very effective cleanser and balancer for the lowest energy center, termed the survival (base) chakra. The person in need of Trilliurn has a disproportionate amount of energy directed towards attaining personal power and wealth.

This excessive concern for personal welfare dominates over all other more altruistic feelings. Such a person easily falls prey to the forces of materialism and greed, feeling the need for many possessions and other forms of material wealth and power. Trillium may also be suitable for those who are poor but believe that the acquisition of wealth and power brings fulfillment. This imbalance of the soul can also be reflected in the body, especially when the body retains too much matter and does not eliminate enough toxins.

At the deepest level, such individuals are disconnected from their spiritual strength; they try to overcome the unconscious sense of helplessness by exercising social and material power. Since their awareness is limited to the physical plane, such individuals can measure their self-worth only with a material yardstick.

Trillium encourages these individuals to shift their awareness to a level beyond the personal, to derive a sense of personal well-being from the relationship with the higher power.

Once the forces held in the lower chakra are purified and released, such people will have a great ability to take possession of the spiritual forces and make them available to others and to the Earth..

Australian flowers for the fourth chakra

The Australian Bush Flowers are today 69 plus 19 essences created by the combination of Australian Flowers and were introduced by Ian White, Australian biologist and psychologist. They are not yet well known and used in Italy by the general public, but they are highly appreciated by flower therapists and we find Australian flowers included in many herbal and homeopathic complexes. They are among the most powerful and widely used flowers after Bach Flowers, they have a very high energy, one of the highest among floral remedies. Australian Aborigines have always used Flowers to treat discomfort or emotional imbalances, as was the case in ancient Egypt, India, Asia and South America.

The dose, for both adults and children, consists of seven drops to be taken twice a day (morning and evening) under the tongue, or in a little water. The essences should be taken for about twenty days or a month, except for particularly powerful essences.

Being a completely natural and non-toxic cure, they have no contraindications, do not cause side effects, can be combined without problems with both traditional and homeopathic medicines (of which they are considered complementary) or other flower therapy remedies. You can prepare a single remedy (whose action will then be particularly "targeted", deep and fast), or mix different remedies together; in this case it is advisable not to exceed 4 or 5 essences and, if possible, try to choose flowers with similar and synergistic properties to treat a specific problem.

Australian flowers are also very effective when applied to the skin and can be added to creams, gels, massage oils, medicated ointments or diluted in bath water. For a topical treatment, the recommended quantity is about 7 drops of each chosen remedy, to be mixed in half a cup of cream; instead, 15–20 drops of each essence should be poured into the bathtub.

The duration of treatment always depends on the individual response. A positive reaction is often obtained in about two weeks and on average two months are sufficient to rebalance numerous psychophysical problems. Some particularly "powerful" flowers (such as, for example, Waratah) usually exert a very rapid action, even in a few days. Many times, after resolving an inner discomfort or conflict, other emotional imbalances can emerge, which will gradually be treated with the corresponding flowers.

Illawara Flame Tree

It is indicated for those people who feel rejected, left out, not loved.

For those who ignore their potential and are afraid of responsibilities. They are people who know what they have to do, but feel burdened by the responsibility of doing it. The flower gives self-acceptance, self-confidence and inner strength.

When rejection, imaginary or real, is manifested, the person is deeply hurt, with a feeling of abandonment. To avoid possible rejection they do things they don't want to do. They know they possess certain skills, but are unable to develop or exploit them.

They ignore their own potentials, making themselves exempt from the responsibility of applying them to themselves.

The essence helps to take the first step towards the realization of one's potential, it makes one become familiar with the true aspirations of life without feeling crushed by responsibility.

They are people who also tend to reject themselves, sometimes falling into a state of depression.

Excellent for children because it can be of help in situations of exclusion, such as from the football team or from the dominant group or who are placed in a new school where, if teachers and classmates do not pay much attention to them, they experience this situation as a rejection and instead of trying to make friends, they get discouraged.

These subjects are characterized by a particular psychological feature in which self-marginalization, suffering in the face of rejection and fear of responsibility form the central structure of the picture. Another characteristic trait is intense apprehension of new situations or experiences. Without a doubt, these personalities are very insecure and constantly need to be loved and accepted. They suffer a lot from being left out of a situation, whether it's brought about by something extreme or just simply an irrelevant fact of life that no other person would care about. Both the apprehensive behavior and the fear of exclusion lead them to develop prejudiced behavior with people, although in reality this attitude is a defense against the deep pain caused by emotional disappointments, abuses and the lack of being taken into consideration.

The main function of this essence is to give confidence, the ability to compromise, internal strength, self-approval. It helps to face the first step in new situations and takes away the fear of exclusion and rejection. This flower works very well in situations where there are difficulties and fears in taking on new responsibilities, such as fatherhood, marriage, etc.

Also useful in menopause where one can feel devalued, with the feeling of not being desirable and therefore being rejected.

Bach flowers for the fourth chakra

Bach flowers are an alternative medicine created by the British doctor Edward Bach, born on 24 September 1886 in Moseley from a Welsh family in England. He graduated in medicine in 1912 and immediately worked in the emergency room of the university hospital where he began to be noticed for the large amount of time he devoted to patients. He was immediately critical of other doctors, who studied the disease as if it were separate from the individual, without focusing on the patients themselves.

It is well known that our emotional states have a profound influence on our well-being and health. An altered emotional state that repeats itself every day creates real dysfunctions in our body.

Ninety per cent of the causes of human disease come from planes beyond the physical, and it is on these planes that symptoms begin to manifest before the physical body shows any disturbance. If we can identify the negative moods that crop up when we get sick, we can fight the disease better and heal faster. Using floral remedies you try to influence the deeper structures from which the disease originates. Bach flowers rebalance the emotions. They address only and exclusively how we react emotionally to the vicissitudes, experiences and problems in our days. They give great serenity and peace, courage or strength, they help us feel at the fullest of our possibilities.

They can be useful in the face of an illness, not from a physical point of view but just as a mood support. The person is seen as a complete individual where emotions are a pivotal point, and not just as a physical body with symptoms. It is therefore necessary to analyze the emotional state and not the physical symptoms, based on this the suitable remedies are found. In fact subjects with identical physical problems react and live with different emotions and feelings. Bach flowers have no contraindications and do not interact with medicines.

Bach has thus divided the 38 flowers from which the remedies are drawn. The very first flowers discovered by Bach were the so-called "12 Healers", which the Welsh doctor promptly began to experiment first on himself and then on his patients; the other 26 were discovered a short time later, divided into "7 Helpers" and "19 Assistants".

Dr Bach later abandoned the distinction between 'Healers', 'Helpers' and 'Assistants' as superfluous, but many people around the world still use it. Bach Flowers do not help to repress negative attitudes, but transform them into their positive side. The Bach Flowers associated with the first chakra are only in general, because the flowers must still be chosen based on the emotion that is not in harmony and must be balanced.

Agrimony

It belongs to the category of "Healers".

Agrimony is for all those who are afraid to show their feelings, always smiling, often wear the mask of cheerful people, even when they suffer. They use stimulants when they have problems nagging them.

In Agrimony the tension, internal anxiety is not manifested with others. What worries is kept hidden and masked with the desire to laugh at all costs. Sometimes Agrimony-type people use alcohol or stimulants to try to maintain this facade of serenity. They usually dislike loneliness, finding it more difficult to wear this mask when alone with themselves.

On the contrary, they always try to surround themselves with friends, parties and blinding lights. However, at night, when they find themselves alone with their thoughts, that mental torture that they had managed to repress so well comes back to haunt them inexorably. The Agrimony remedy helps people who have such a character trait to accept the darker sides of life and of their personality and come to terms with them, so that they become more complete human beings, without losing their sense of humour, but being able to laugh at one's problems to solve them rather than hide them.

Moods and symptoms related to Agrimony in order of importance:

- Forced cheerfulness
- Anxiety hidden by cheerfulness

- Anxiety and fear
- Anxiety for which you eat even at night
- Tendency to avoid discussions
- Anxiety localized in the chest
- Nervous hunger
- Hidden inner conflicts
- Fear of discussions
- Tightness in the chest
- They bite their nails
- Teeth grinding in sleep

To prepare the floral remedy, the flowers that have just opened or in bud are picked, before bees or other insects have visited them, and are prepared with the sun method between June and August.

Centaury

It belongs to the category of "Healers".

Centaury is the remedy for people who find it difficult to say no to others. They are good-natured and kind and love to help others. Sometimes, however, unscrupulous people take advantage of it and the individual Centaury finds himself, in spite of himself, a slave to the desires and will of others. The Centaury remedy does not numb the Centaury personality, but rather helps this type of person develop courage and self-determination so as to be able to say enough at the right time and not submit to the wishes and orders of others.

The lack of ability to impose one's own opinions and needs makes one weak, even physically. Often one is a Red Cross nurse and behind this great desire to help others hides one's inability to assert oneself and then complain that one feels exploited. This state of mind can arise in various situations: towards a child, towards a partner, a parent, or as a weakness towards a vice: such as cigarettes, sweets, food, expensive clothes, luxury cars, drugs, gambling, sex.

The essence helps the will and self-respect, gives energy, allows to be able to affirm one's personality and to have a balanced attitude towards others, gives the ability to give but without being overwhelmed. The new self-determination will restore vitality and zest for life.

With Centaury you know your values and your needs. You are capable of integrating with others, but respecting your own uniqueness.

The person with this disposition will gain energy, become more determined and will be able to express his opinion when necessary.

Centaury-related moods and symptoms in order of importance:

- You are not able to say no, even to food in cases of nervous hunger
- Need for confirmation from others with excessive availability towards others
- Excess of love that makes you forget your own interests
- Exaggerated concern for the good of others
- Altruism that leads to feeling exploited
- Altruism as self-denial
- Low esteem because you tend to serve others
- Anxiety to please others
- Lack of decision-making power
- Indulge others
- Desire for pleasure
- Fear of discussions
- Exaggerated altruism
- Shyness with little individuality

The preparation for the floral remedy follows the sun method, taking care to pick the inflorescences (without touching them) from as many plants as possible and then placing them in a basin of pure water until the surface is covered.

Between May and September it has star-shaped flowers with five petals, with a tube-shaped corolla and in pink or red bunches. The harvest takes place from June to August.

Holly

It belongs to the category of "Assistants".

Whoever needs this flower is a person who gets angry easily, yells, offends and is aggressive, snaps violently at anything and this can happen anywhere: in a bar, restaurant, car, on the street; he always overreacts to the circumstance. In the ultra negative state, in addition to getting angry easily, he completely loses the light of reason by breaking anything, for example if the computer gives problems it is also capable of destroying it, in short, he lashes out at anything only because he cannot react and when he is wronged by a person throws himself at him like a fury.

Holly's "negative" state blocks oneself and sees the outside world only as a source of cheating against ourselves, creating hatred and jealousy.

Holly allows you to relax by opening up with trust towards others. The person with this disposition will be more peaceful, the floral remedy calms and no longer makes one lose the light of reason so easily; she turns anger into love. With Holly you live in love, without tension but with the clarity and understanding necessary to love.

Holly is often thought of as the Anger Fix, but that's not necessarily the case. The Holly remedy is used for anger when it is accompanied by hatred, suspicion, envy or jealousy. In other cases of anger, other remedies are needed, such as Impatiens, when the anger is caused by impatience, Vervain, when it is caused by a sense of injustice, or Chicory when the person is angry because he feels offended and hurt by the anger. ingratitude of others.

Holly-related moods and symptoms in order of importance:

- Morbid jealousy
- Rancor with hatred
- Grudge
- Absence of love towards one's neighbor
- Manifest envy
- Joy for the problems of others
- Anger with hatred
- Revenge
- Cruelty to others
- Aggression due to jealousy
- Bitterness due to disappointment
- Absence of love that leads to feeling alone
- Expressed anger

The floral remedy is prepared with the boiling method, using the tops of the branches with both male and female flowers and some new leaves.

Walnut

It belongs to the category of "Assistants".

Whoever needs this flower is in a life-changing situation or is in a condition in which they do not have the strength to change, such as: marriage, divorce, new job, climate change, retirement, menopause, bereavement, pregnancy, vacation, new partner. Taking Walnut when experiencing a change facilitates adaptation by discovering new resources to easily experience the new situation. It is also useful for those who are sensitive to the tensions of their surroundings and who tend to make them their own. Also indicated for those suffering from meteoropathy (symptoms related to meteorological factors). Walnut helps break ties with the past, thus allowing you to continue on your path with confidence and without excessive suffering. With Walnut you are protected in changes, you feel safe and each new phase is lived with ease.

Walnut-related moods and symptoms in order of importance:

- To facilitate any kind of change
- Menopause
- Hypersensitive to changes
- Stages of change
- Puberty

Number of the third chakra

12 is the number of the fourth chakra.

It is considered the holiest of numbers, along with three and seven.

The twelve is closely related to the three, since its reduction is equivalent to this number ($12 = 1 + 2 = 3$) and since it is given by the multiplication of 3 by 4.

- Three is the number that represents the relationship between Wisdom, Power and Love. This balance is the primary focus of the Heart Chakra. Wisdom without Love and Power would be cruel and weak.
- Power without Wisdom and Love would be dangerous and selfish.
- Love without Power and Wisdom would be victimized and stupid.

In our hearts we must learn how to find and unite all three of these virtues.

Twelve was very significant in ancient human life due to the fact of the twelve tribes of Israel, the twelve disciples who followed Jesus, the twelve signs of the zodiac and the twelve hours into which a clock is divided. The Twelve has a very marked esoteric meaning as it is associated with the physical and mystical tests that the initiate must complete. Passing the tests leads to a transformation, as the passage takes place on difficult tests, the only ones that lead to real growth. In many cultures the initiatory rites are performed at the age of twelve, after which one enters adulthood. Most ancient number and measurement systems were based on Twelve, examples being the dozen, the shilling (12p) and the foot (which measures 12 inches).

It is a sublime number; in mathematics, a sublime number is a positive integer that has a perfect number of positive divisors (including itself), and whose positive divisors can add up to get another perfect number.

The number 12 is a sublime number as it has a perfect number of positive divisors (6): 1, 2, 3, 4, 6, and 12, and the sum of these again gives a perfect number:

$1 + 2 + 3 + 4 + 6 + 12 = 28.$

This number undoubtedly has great importance in the texts of the Holy Scriptures and also for Israel. Twelve contains a great symbolic value, not only because it implies its spatio-temporal origin, probably derived from other cultures such as the Babylonian one (in which, for example, the number represented the universe in its internal complexity: the duodenum which characterizes the year, and the zodiac; twelve indicates the fullness of the year, made up of twelve months), but also and above all because it represents the number of the election, that of the people of God.

The twelve sons of Israel-Jacob are the eponymous ancestors of the twelve tribes of Israel. Furthermore, in the book of Numbers, we read that dedication offerings were presented at the altar, beginning on the day it was anointed (that is, consecrated): each day that followed, until the twelfth, an offering was presented from part of a representative of each of the tribes of Israel.

Phisical exercises

- **Exercise 1**

Do some relaxation exercises by shaking your arms and legs.
Sit on the floor with your back straight and then do alternate breathing for a few minutes.

- **Exercise 2**

Assume the quadruped position and perform the "horse's back / cat's arched back" exercise 7 times.

- **Exercise 3**

Lie on your stomach, with your forehead in contact with the ground, arms alongside your body.
Then cross your hands behind your back at the height of the buttocks.
Inhaling, lift your head and sternum slightly and bring your shoulders back a little so that the sternum is relaxed.
From this position breathe deeply 2 times then release the tension.
Repeat the exercise 3 times.

- **Exercise 4**

The finger placement for this breathing exercise is different for men and women.

Women connect the thumb and ring finger of the left hand and the thumb and middle finger of the right hand, men vice versa.

Close your eyes and relax, inhale and exhale pronounce the mantra "yam".

Repeat the exercise 7 times focusing on the heart chakra.

- **Exercise 5**

Lie on your back, close your eyes, place your hands palms down on your heart, right over left.

Breathe deeper and deeper imagining that you are receiving the energy of the cosmos as you inhale and making it flow through the center of your chest as you exhale.

Imagine the light green colored energy, feeling it radiating throughout your body as it enters from the heart.

Repeat at least 7 breathing cycles, then lower your hands to the ground and relax.

Stones for the 4th Chakra

In crystallotherapy, stones of the 4th Chakra are considered those whose color is green and pink.

In crystallotherapy we consider two different work areas, depending on whether we intervene to free from repressed pain or whether we act to develop the ability to love, from the human to the spiritual level.

In the first case, green colored stones of any type of luster or transparency are used.

The most representative basic frequency stone is Aventurine, while the most representative advanced frequency stone is Chrysoprase.

In this case the location of the stones is the base of the sternum or the diaphragm, where the ribs widen and the abdominal cavity begins.

If, on the other hand, one acts to develop the ability to love, the most representative basic frequency stone is Rose Quartz, while the most representative advanced frequency stone is Kunzite. In this case the placement area of the stones is the center of the chest, at heart level.

Crystals that can balance the second chakra are amazonite, aventurine, chalcedony, green calcite, rose quartz, emerald, malachite, green spinel, green tourmaline, unakite kunzite.

Feel its energy passing through the sacral chakra as you hold it in your hand or wear it by ring or necklace.

You don't have to buy them all, just choose the stones you prefer or which you already have.

Amazonite

It is not clear where the name comes from the amazonite stone. Some sources say that the term amazonite derives from the name of the Amazon River, even if no deposits have ever been found there, others instead argue that its name is in honor of mythical female warriors, the Amazons, whose favorite color was the green. Amazonite properties are used for artistic creativity and energy healing.

It is an excellent stone for communication, trust and leadership. Reduces self-harming behaviors, increases self-respect, grace, self-confidence with external communication.

The benefits of amazonite are calming to the brain and nervous system, helping to filter information and combine it with natural intuition to enhance understanding, and to enhance one's ability to cooperate with others, as well as the ability to express oneself. themselves.

Amazonite is connected with material energies.

Excellent stone for protection of one's home and environmental energies, and for the energy strengthening of objects or talismans. It is suggested to use Amazonite in combination with Atlantisite, Jade and Chalcopyrite. Considered a lucky stone, especially by players, Amazonite has the great ability to calm the mood swings of the soul, thus acting as a tranquilizer. It also greatly increases decision-making power, making the person who wears it safer and free from fears from the outside world. This is why it instills a strong sense of security and at the same time helps to cultivate a deep and persistent spirit of trust both in oneself and in others.

The consequence of this is the great facility to create and lead intense interpersonal relationships.

Amazonite, in practice, gives a strong balance to Yin and Yang energies. Its therapeutic faculties are many: suitable for relieving sore throats and diseases of the respiratory tract in general; it is well suited to pregnant women and to those who, due to daily stress, experience the first symptoms of a nervous breakdown.

But its properties don't end there: it has muscle-relaxing properties, especially after making great efforts, it helps the liver to metabolize foods that are difficult to absorb and, in general, it helps relax the whole body, relieving the sense of tiredness.

At the endocrine and hormonal level, it harmonizes the functions of the pituitary gland and the thymus, while at the neuronal level, it regulates the vegetative system.

According to an ancient legend, handed down by the Indios of the Amazon, this stone came from a place called "Land of Women".

Even today, in fact, it is believed that Amazonite has the ability to make the women who wear it more beautiful and attractive.

Aventurine

Its name means "ventura" (by chance) deriving from a very similar glass discovered by chance, in fact, in the eighteenth century in the city of Venice. Aventurine has been used for several centuries in the making of jewellery, vases and other ornamental pieces. They were found in the Omo valley in Ethiopia, primitive tools of aventurine used as points and axes, dated about 2 million years.

Green aventurine is comparable to the lucky four-leaf clover: it is often placed in bags to keep close to bring abundance and good luck in money. Aventurine is also used in spells and ritual magic.

The stone has the ability to enhance its user's sense of humor and gaiety. It's also an excellent balancing stone, it gives inner balance and stimulates dreams. It has a positive effect on the psyche, reinforcing a sense of individualism, and is the ideal stone for those seeking a positive outlook on life.

Aventurine is useful in ailments of the lungs, sinus and heart, and to help increase muscle flexibility.

It can help balance the innermost and dormant emotions (great combination with malachite) and is one of the best stones to wear or carry during times of stress. It is also historically known for being able to bring out the heat of fever and inflammation.

If we use more aventurine stones in the bath water, they become stones for calming emotional pain and fears, managing to dissolve blockages in the heart chakra. On the spiritual side, Aventurine is an excellent aid in understanding where our life is moving and what choices we must make to pursue our true path.

The corresponding Chakra is the 4th, that of the Heart.

As for Green Aventurine, its properties are more calming and aimed at the nervous system; it acts excellently on tachycardia and stress and is a good remedy for skin pathologies due to nervous problems.

The zodiac signs associated with this variety are Taurus, Cancer and Sagittarius.

Rose Quartz

The wrought rose quartz stone has been found in the area once known as Mesopotamia (present day Iraq) with pieces dating back to 6000 BC.

Rose quartz jewelry was made by the Assyrians during the time frame of 800 - 600 BC, and it is believed that the Assyrians together with the Romans were the first to use this stone as objects for esoteric or divination purposes. The Romans also used it to make seals as a sign of ownership. The Egyptians believed that, if worn, it would prevent aging.

- Rose quartz works closely with the Heart chakra and is, in fact, called the Heart Stone: it represents love, beauty, peace, and forgiveness. Excellent stone to use for meditations by placing it on the heart chakra and imagining that, through the breath, its sweet pink light spreads love, serenity and well-being in us.

It is a sweet, gentle stone, a calming stone that warms the center of our heart. It is able to balance our emotions, thus giving inner peace and harmony. Rose Quartz energy is among the most relaxing and promotes empathy, reconciliation and forgiveness of others.

It is able to reduce stress and tension in the heart, eliminate anger, jealousy and resentment in others, relieving heart problems and discomfort associated with holding such negative emotions in us. Rose Quartz helps us understand that all changes in our lives are important, even the most difficult changes to accept.

- Rose Quartz can also be used to balance all chakras and to remove inharmonious energy and replace it with love energy.

He is capable of aligning the mental, emotional and astral bodies on his own, which is why it is always useful to carry stones or wear some jewellery. A quick way to benefit from the sensual and loving virtues of rose quartz is to drink a spring water elixir with the essence of the stone.

Furthermore, to promote a calm and harmonious environment where we live, it is very advisable to have at least one piece or several pieces scattered in strategic places, such as desks, bedside tables or shelves..

Emerald

Emerald stones are among the most appreciated: the green energy, which vibrates with the heart chakra, makes the mineral the stone of success and abundance. To encourage the removal of negativity, tradition has it that natural emerald crystals are able to stimulate positive actions and results, providing the strength to overcome any problems in life.

The light green color is present in nature in grass, plants and trees, which give off the energy just mentioned. The force of nature is always enclosed in green minerals, exactly as in the case of the emerald.

This stone also has many excellent qualities and is usually associated with those born in the month of May.

It is commonly used in engagement rings as it carries strong loving vibrations.

The name derives from the Greek, precisely "green stone". Emeralds are a variety of beryl: very popular for jewellery, they come mostly from India, Russia, Zimbabwe, Africa, Egypt, Austria, Brazil and Colombia. The green ray of these beautiful stones encourages you to have respect for all life forms and for all of creation, living with more love.

All emerald specimens emit this energy and have a strong effect on the deepest emotions. Feelings such as compassion, hope, loyalty, reassurance, kindness, benevolence, goodness and unconditional love are connected to a cosmic and spiritual form of love, which embraces every living being.

For those who believe in the potential of stones and crystal healing, all people are "Divine Beings in a physical body". Yet many feel blocks in living a life full and characterized by love. Stress leads to brooding over one's misfortunes every day; meditating with the emerald can help you improve, rediscovering yourself full of love for yourself and for others. Additionally, these stones can soothe negative e motions and create positive vibes, to help you break through the psychological obstacles that block energy potentials.

Emerald is also used to relieve stress, improve memory and facilitate understanding. It can also stimulate economic abundance.

A new prosperity at all levels can be the natural result of being accompanied by the emerald and its energy. Carrying an emerald in your pocket during the day and keeping it under your pillow at night can already be very useful, not to mention that jewels with emerald stones or gems are all very beautiful and elegant. The longer the emerald is kept in one's aura, the more benefits it can produce within the wearer.

It is possible to combine emerald with other varieties of beryl, such as aquamarine and goshenite.

Moreover:

- Pale green hyddenite has a strong energy that combines well with emerald to aid in emotional healing. For this purpose, other stones that can be combined are green apophyllite, pink rhodochrosite, rhodonite and lilac lepidolite.

- Among the stones that can be used with the emerald, there are others that vibrate with the heart chakra, such as dioptase, green aventurine, green amethyst, variscite and moldavite. Again, pink kunzite, pink quartz and pink morganite of the same color.

Malachite

Malachite owes its name to the belief from the Greek word "Malache" which means "mallow" (a green herb).

The properties of malachite are thought to be able to reach the innermost feelings of the person and reflect who one is, negative or positive. In fact, malachite is called the "mirror stone of the soul".

Malachite has been believed since ancient times to be a powerful protector of children, and it is believed to protect the wearer from accidents. It protects travelers and is of strong balance in relationships. Malachite powder was already used as early as 3000 BC. by the ancient Egyptians as a cosmetic for eye make-up.

It is believed that looking at or wearing malachite can relax the nervous system and calm emotional turmoil, bringing a sense of peace and harmony.

Malachite reminds us that we have a dual nature, and it is the job of each person to know and govern their person.

To be used combined with copper to increase its power.

Green Tourmaline

Stimulates the joy of living, emphasizing all the positive aspects of life. It makes us open and patient, soliciting interest in others.

Promotes creativity and positive thinking.

It restores balance, giving great energy and versatility. It enhances the ability to plan and helps to achieve one's goals.

Relieves the sense of tiredness and promotes the regeneration of nerves torn by stress.

- Has a beneficial effect on the heart and acts as a detoxifier. Placed on the cardiac plexus of the fourth chakra, it cures all diseases of viral origin, even the most serious, by regulating the functionality of the thymus and blood pressure (both too high and too low). Increase awareness by acting directly on the heart chakra.

Balances emotions and opens our soul to love. This is why it is good to use it together with Rose Quartz.

Strengthens the central nervous system, the immune system and the entire respiratory system. Stimulates the joy of living, makes you open to others and patient. It would act on the nervous system by purifying it, increasing its ability to convey energy and balancing the two cerebral hemispheres. Gives resistance to stress and tiredness.

Unakite

Unakite stone gets its name from the Greek word "epidosis" which means "to grow together".

This name is due to the fact that unakite is the result of three minerals together: feldspar, epidote and quartz, and it is precisely through these materials joined together that unakite conveys its particular message. It is a stone that balances our emotional and spiritual bodies, providing us with an extremely gentle release of our energy blockages anchored in the solar plexus.

It helps us overcome the outdated beliefs of the past and facilitates the understanding of previous events and their importance in our growth path. It keeps our spirits up when we are feeling low or easily conditioned, never letting us lose sight of the beauty of life.

It is useful for the reproductive system, for healthy pregnancies and for the healthy and harmonious development of unborn children.

Also used during recovery from major trauma, it helps us by prompting our body to remember the state of perfect health.

Carrying it will help us maintain a healthy balance between the spiritual and mundane lives, allowing them to communicate in order to help us create the life we need.

In addition to helping bring us back to earth, it drives away, through meditations, the pain and anger that are often sedimented in us and that we find it hard to let go.

- Excellent combination with moonstone, unakite helps to keep the connection between the lower chakras and the upper chakras firmly through the heart chakra. It can also, over time, build and entrench self-confidence, strengthening our inner courage, helping us take control of those aspects of our lives that can produce power.

Kunzite

It awakens the heart and unconditional love, generating benevolent thoughts and serene communication. Radiate peace and connect to universal love. Kunzite induces a deep meditative state and is beneficial for those who find it difficult to enter meditation.

Promotes creativity, encourages humility and a willingness to serve others. Kunzite is a protective stone, which acts on the individual and the environment and has the power to disperse negativity. This stone shields the aura from unwanted energies, creating a protective envelope around it and removing the entities that have implanted themselves in it, as well as mental influences. Kunzite allows you to contain yourself, even in a crowd, and strengthens the energy field around the body.

Encourages free expression of ego and feelings. It facilitates the individual journey, freeing it from any obstacles and favoring adaptation to the constant pressures of life. It can help recover memories that seemed repressed and is a useful therapy for people who have grown up too fast, allowing them to regain their lost trust and innocence. It induces tolerance towards oneself and others, and is recommended for reducing the stress caused by anxiety.

Kunzite facilitates introspection and the ability to act critically and constructively. It has the power to combine intellect, intuition and inspiration. It can be used to shed light on emotional fragments and release emotions, especially healing anguish, a legacy of previous lives. It overcomes resistance and helps to reach compromises between one's own needs and those of others. The property of kunzite to improve mood is a good antidote against depression of emotional origin and is excellent for relieving panic attacks.

- It activates the heart chakra and aligns it with the throat and third eye. This stone strengthens the circulatory system and heart muscle. It is useful for affections of a nervous nature, such as neuralgia. Calms epilepsy and relieves joint pain. Neutralizes the effects of anesthesia and stimulates the immune system. Kunzite contains lithium, for this reason it will prove effective for psychiatric disorders and depression, especially if taken in the form of an elixir.

Green Agate

The green agate gemstone meaning is associated with health, abundance, and good fortune. It is a symbol of fertility and can be used in spells to create a bountiful garden or a bountiful harvest.

Green agate has healing powers to help the heart, blood vessels and circulatory system. It can also help detoxify the body and strengthen the immune system.

Agates get their name from the ancient Greek city of Achates, which was located on the island of Sicily, according to Geology.com.

Agate is a member of the quartz family, a group of minerals that includes amethyst and citrine.

The quartz family takes its name from the word "quartz", which means hard rock or crystal. Quartz is one of the most abundant minerals in the world, making up about 12% of all minerals found in the earth's crust.

This crystal is one of the best for relaxation and stress recovery. Promotes good sleep and allows you to wake up cheerful and full of energy. The stone helps to gain self-confidence, relieve depression, fear, panic attacks and negative emotions. Green agate increases physical strength, reduces tiredness and muscle pain after intense exercise or heavy physical effort. This mineral calms the nervous system and relieves blockages in the spine. Green agate is useful for people who have vision problems. This crystal is also good for people who often get sore throats or hoarseness.

Green agate is recommended for women with hormonal imbalances. It can be used as a talisman during pregnancy: it will help calm the mother when she feels bad or gets scared about something.

- Green agate can help maintain heart health and keep it functioning properly, so it is highly recommended for those who have problems with heart health.

Moldavite

It is commonly referred to as moldavite stone, but in reality it is a natural glassy substance (from the tektite group) of a transparent bottle-green color whose formation dates back to 15 million years ago following the fall of a huge meteorite in the region of the current Czech Republic The shards of molten rock following the impact cooled in flight and scattered up to 400 km away in the territory of the Vltava river from which this material takes its name. In short, a crystal that comes from space.

Moldavite speeds up the healing process and is helpful in diagnosing diseases. It is particularly suitable for flu states with fever and cough, asthma and bronchitis.

The effects of moldavite in the purification processes on the energy centers of the body can manifest themselves with temporary tingling and dizziness.

Moldavite opens the mind to higher levels of knowledge, accelerates and amplifies the spirituality of the individual. With her feminine energy she removes blocks in all chakras, especially those involving the fourth, strengthens the ability to identify with others and communicate with spiritual guides.

Moldavite is a stone of change: it helps to free the individual from the conditionings of material reality, such as worries related to money and the future, brings out dreams and memories that open to understanding the meaning of one's existence and stimulates more creative solutions to problems.

On a physical level it is a good stone when it comes to supporting a healing process in general. In this sense it can be combined with other stones, based on what your problem is.

- Wear a moldavite pendant to see beyond your horizons, learn how to find the solution to problems you can't figure out.
- Bring it into contact with the skin or if you want to use it in a crystal therapy session, put it in contact with the heart chakra or with the third eye (when you need to bring back memories).
- If you want to bring a dash of creativity into your work, bring a moldavite as a pendant, bracelet or simply place one on your desk.

Olivine

Olivine, sometimes called peridot, is a crystal with remarkable properties.

Olivine is connected to the heart chakra and is in strong harmony with the earth element. As the name suggests, it has a very bright green color (some may appear yellow or brownish) and is semi-transparent. However, there is also a yellow note inside, which differentiates it for example from malachite which has a blue note. This color makes olivine also suitable for working on the solar plexus and allows you to work on physical vibrations and restore harmony.

Use it to bring clarity and open your mind to different levels of awareness. It helps you to grow, to recognize your destiny and your true path.

You can use olivine to stimulate the heart chakra. In this way you can intervene on your way of interacting with others and thus unlock various behaviors that make you feel uncomfortable with other people but also with the environment.

It helps you if you feel controlled within the relationship, if you are critical of others and always try to find another weakness in order to infer. It helps you to be in balance, increase empathy and better understand others.

However, peridot also contains a hint of yellow inside, so you can use it for the third chakra.

Manipura governs relationships, helps you balance yourself and counteract fear. Place it on the solar plexus to release nervous tension, guilt and anxiety.

www.ingramcontent.com/pod-product-compliance
Lightning Source LLC
Chambersburg PA
CBHW050534280326
41933CB00011B/1588